CW00470761

Artificial Insemination On A Budget - Our Tips & Tricks For A Successful At Home Insemination

By Sarah Jane Correia and Emma L Jackson

The Fine Print

Forward

After the publication of our first book on artificial insemination at home, <u>Lesbian Pregnancy On A Budget : Two Moms' Tale Of Having A Baby</u>, we were contacted by a number of our readers. They shared with us a fact that we had overlooked - the information we discussed would be quite helpful to single women and heterosexual couples who were struggling to conceive their own children due to the cost of traditional AI attempts. This book is a revised version of our methods, taking into account the different types of needs and issues that these types of potential parents may face.

Our story is not that different to a lot of those parents-to-be out there. I was a healthy woman who wanted to get pregnant. My partner Emma (being another woman) couldn't get me pregnant. Because I had no medical issues myself that prevented me from conceiving a child, I was not eligible for any kind of insurance coverage to help offset the costs of "professional" artificial insemination. I certainly wasn't going to have sex with a man I didn't care about just to get pregnant. (Besides the obvious, we didn't want to have any issues about custody of our future child in the event the man discovered he had conceived a child - knowingly or unknowingly.) Of course, we could have attempted to fund the artificial insemination treatments ourselves, but the fact that at hundreds of dollars a try, and more than likely needing multiple tries to get pregnant, we simply couldn't afford it.

That's when the year of research began. Through our research, talking with other couples, and good old fashioned trial and error, we managed to find a way for me to get pregnant without breaking the budget. All all, we spent less than a few hundred dollars, and were able to conceive a child the first time we put our final plan to task. That's not to say that we had many 'draft' plans, and unsuccessful plans, but we found the one that worked for us, and that will hopefully work for you as well.

I became pregnant in February of 2010, and after a healthy pregnancy we were blessed with our son in November 2010. We hope that our readers will be able to use the knowledge we have collected to have their own blessings without the worry of being able to get pregnant on a budget.

-Sarah Jane

Table of Contents

The Biology of Pregnancy – A Quick Sex Ed Refresher

In order to get pregnant in the first place, you need to know how it all works. The first steps we took was to remind ourselves of those things that we learned in those embarrassing classes of our youth – what the female menstrual cycle was all about, when it's physically possible to get pregnant, and how exactly fertilization happens.

Let's break down the parts of a menstrual cycle, shall we?

Phase Name	Description	Start Day (Assuming 28 day cycle)	Average End Day
Menstrual Phase	When the bleeding occurs, due to the body shedding the uterine lining.	1	4
Proliferate Phase	When the body starts replacing the uterine lining.	5	13
Ovulation	When the ovaries release an egg, and the egg travels down the fallopian tubes.	13	16
Luteal Phase	When the body is getting ready for the next menstrual phase, when implantation occurs.	16	28

The menstrual cycle is what enables ladies to have their babies. If you don't have a cycle, or have a very irregular cycle, it makes it very difficult to get pregnant.

Unlike what our high-school sex ed teachers told us in school, the chances of getting pregnant any day of your cycle are pretty slim. We learned that there are days where you have a greater chance of getting pregnant, and days where you have a less chance. For us, we concentrated on ovulation, when Sarah had the greatest chance of getting pregnant, which is typically day 14 of a 28 day cycle.

Now, keep in mind that this is what the textbook case is. In our case, Sarah wasn't textbook. So how can you figure out when exactly you are going to ovulate, and time that insemination so that it coincides with your most fertile time? I'll go over that in greater detail in another chapter.

That's the ladies end of the biology. Now for the man's – or at least the part that's important to us.

Sperm 'swim' through the cervical fluid in a woman's body, hopefully making its way to an awaiting egg for insemination. It only takes a single sperm to fertilize an egg, which is key to remember when you look at the small 'deposit' that your donor has provided and have the dread that there's not enough there. In this case, a little does go a long way. When our donor handed us a vial of what looked like a teaspoon of seminal fluid, we audibly gasped, only to calm ourselves later with that information.

here are certain things your donor can do to increase their sperm count, and things that you can do to create an atmosphere in your uterus that is more habitable for the sperm. We'll go over those later on as well.

ght. Enough middle school biology.

Preparing for Pregnancy – A Collection of Methods to Determine Ovulation

If we were to give one piece of advice to any woman hoping to get pregnant, is to track your cycle in as many ways as possible. We also strongly suggest you join an online fertility tracking site. While there are many that you can pay for, there are also perfectly good free ones. We used Fertility Friend which is free and quite detailed.

Some may question why we chose to go into this section in such detail. Our answer is that unless you know your body, you are wasting valuable time (and sometimes money). Below, we've listed methods you can use to determine your ovulation, tools that we used when using this process, and our opinion of the method in general.

Date Tracking Method – This method uses patterns in your cycle to estimate when you are ovulating, based on the start date of your period on previous cycles. After several months of tracking, you establish your longest and shortest cycle. To determine the start fertile time, you subtract 18 from the length of your shortest cycle. The end of your fertile time is calculated by subtracting 11 from the length of your longest cycle.

For example, if your shortest cycle was 27 days long, your fertile time start day would be day 9. If your longest cycle was 33 days long, the end of your fertile time is day 22. Somewhere between day and day 22, you will ovulate.

you are using an online tracker, the math is done for you.

Cost: Free to a few dollars per month, depending on if you join a paid online tracking site.

Pros: You only update it once a month, when you first get your period. It's quite easy to use if you take advantage of the multiple online trackers available. There are also many apps available for your Kindle, smartphone or tablet. If you are regular, a pattern can emerge quite quickly. There's no mess and little fuss involved.

Cons: It is only an estimation of when you are ovulating, based on previous cycles. It can take several months to establish enough of a pattern to accurately determine when you are ovulating if you aren't regular. It gives you a 'window' of fertility that can be weeks long, and does not narrow down the exact 48 hours of ovulation. No biological factors are taken into account.

What we used: We used Fertility Friend, since it enabled us to also enter other details to more accurately establish when Sarah was ovulating.

What we would use if we tried again: Since Sarah's cycles are 28 days a month without fail, we would give Cyclebeads a try. It uses the same basic concept of counting days, but in a much more tactile method. Rather than filling out charts and tracking on a computer, you slide a ring around a beaded bracelet, and the color of the bead coincides with the dates of your fertile time.

Basal Body Temperature Method: Once your body has released an egg, your body temperature slightly increases, and does not go back down until your next cycle begins. By tracking this chance in temperature, you can use previous months to predict when you will ovulate. For instance, if you see that your body's temperature increases on day 18 of your cycle on a consistent basis, you can assume that you are ovulating around day 16 of your cycle, based on ovulation being 48 hours long.

Cost: $2 to $20+, depending on the type of thermometer purchased

Pros: It's also quite inexpensive. It only takes around a minute each day to complete. It's based on your body's reactions rather than a calendar.

Cons: You have to take your temperature at the exact same time each morning, before you get out of bed (as removing covers can alter your body temperature enough to skew results). This is a bit of a pain if you get up at 7am on the weekdays, and hope for a bit of extra sleep on the weekends. It can take a few months to establish a pattern.

What we used: An ordinary digital oral thermometer that you can get for less than $5, and a printout chart that you can find on the internet.

What we would use if we tried again: We probably would splurge a bit on a digital ear thermometer, just to reduce the amount of time before Sarah could roll over and go back to sleep on a weekend.

Cervical Mucus Method: This is based on the concept that your cervical mucus (abbreviated as CM in a lot of tracking sites) chances as you progress through your cycle. You track the color (clear, white, or cloudy), consistency (thick, sticky or stretchy), and texture (dry, wet, sticky, slippery, stretchy) of the mucus. Typically, the body starts creating mucus around day 8. It goes through several stages until you hit ovulation, when your CM is its clearest, slipperiest, and stretchiest. This is also referred to as 'egg white consistency'. You can print out free trackers online, or you can join ovulation tracking web sites as listed above to document your CM's patterns.

Cost: Free to a few dollars per month, depending on if you join a paid online tracking site.

Pros: This is one of the cheapest ways to track your ovulation directly. It's body-based, not math-based. You can start making assumptions on your ovulation day as soon as your first month.

Cons: If you are not comfortable with your own body fluids, this can be a bit awkward. If you are inseminating, it may be difficult to distinguish between leftover fluids and your CM (as the fluids can still be there days later). You need to wash your hands before retrieving your mucus to avoid any infections.

What we used: The CM tracker that was already included on the Fertility Friend web site.

What we would use if we tried again: Not much you can change here – it's pretty basic as it is!

Cervical Position Method: As your body moves through your monthly cycle, your cervix goes through changes. Using washed hands, you use your fingers to feel inside of your vagina, up to your cervix to determine its position and texture. When you are at your most fertile, your cervix moves higher up into your body, becomes softer, and opens slightly. A low, firm, and closed cervix means that you are generally not fertile. Most online fertility sites let you track cervical positioning.

In our experiences, this didn't work for us. Sarah's cervix was too high to reach, even on her least fertile days. We've listed it here as a method that we tried, and that may be successful for others.

Cost: Free to a few dollars per month, depending on if you join a paid online tracking site.

Pros: Low to no cost, and can be done at any time of the day (but you are best sticking with the same time every day). Your partner can be involved in this process by feeling your cervix for you. I measures changes in your body.

Cons: It's another one of those areas where if you are not comfortable with your own body, this is not something you're likely to want to do. If you've already given birth (including miscarriage), yo cervix may always be open. This is an acquired skill, and not something that's very straight forwar

Ovulation Prediction Kits: Similar to a pregnancy test, these kits test the level of a certain hormone in your urine. When a woman is ovulating, there is an increase in Lutropine (called the LH surge) one to two days before you ovulate. This is the signal that your fertile period has arrived, and it's time to start inseminating. The 12 to 36 hour timeframe between when the levels of Lutropine increase in your body, and when your egg is released is the magic window which has the greatest chance of conception.

There are a variety of products on the market that call themselves ovulation prediction kits. These range from your bargain basement pee-on-a-stick packs, to digital ovulation tests, all the way up to fertility monitors that will set you back three figures.

Cost: $10 to $200, depending on the technology you use

Pros: This is the most exact way to determine your ovulation time.

Cons: Good equipment can be expensive.

What we used: The Clear Blue Easy Fertility Monitor – we became pregnant after our first month of use, and feel that if you are going to 'splurge' on any item we suggest that this be it. We have recommended it to many women over the years, and have many success stories to go along with that.

What we would use if we tried again: We would absolutely use the Clear Blue Easy Fertility Monitor again.

Saliva Ferning Method: This was a concept that neither of us had ever heard of prior to trying to get pregnant. By examining the pattern that your dried saliva makes under a microscope, you can determine when your peak fertility time occurs. When the body is not fertile, the dried saliva resembles small dots. When you are growing more fertile, the saliva starts to crystalize and growing into longer strands. At your peak, the saliva resembles a 'fern', with a long, branching formation. If you've ever seen lines of ice on a frozen windshield, you have a clue what we mean.

The kits to see this ferning are small, lipstick sized microscopes. Some of the more advanced models have lights to illuminate the area. Many fertility tracking web sites allow you to input data from saliva ferning.

Cost: Anywhere from $20 to $200, depending on which type of scope you go for.

Pros: It's quite simple to use. There's minimal mess involved. It's a quick secondary test to add to whatever you are already doing.

Cons: There are some VERY overpriced scopes on the market. A $20 is virtually identical to a $200 scope, with the only difference being magnification power. It's more of a secondary test, rather than something that can stand alone such as fertility monitors or cervical mucus testing.

What we used: Fertile Focus Personal Ovulation Microscope

What we would use if we tried again: If we hadn't passed our scope onto another couple, we'd use it again. But, given the fact that there are so many more reliable methods out there, we probably wouldn't get another scope the next time around.

Finding the Man of Your Dreams – Locating and Connecting with a Sperm Donor

One of the largest costs associated with artificial insemination is the cost of donor sperm. If you're looking at sperm banks, be ready to shell out hundreds of dollars per try. Given the fact that the average woman takes around 3 months to get pregnant, you're looking at more than a thousand dollars in unsuccessful pregnancy attempts.

Fortunately, we didn't pay a single cent for our sperm. No, we didn't use someone we knew, and we don't co-parent with our donor. In fact, we met him twice, and haven't seen him since. This is the arrangement we came to beforehand, as we wanted this experience to mirror a traditional sperm donor experience as possible. So, how do you go about finding a sperm donor, while protecting your and your future child's privacy?

Get A New Email Account - The first thing that we did was create a brand new email address that have no indication of our identity. The email address itself didn't give away any details about us – it didn't include our names, our likes, or resemble other email addresses we had in any way at all. In the fields you fill out where it asks for your first and last name, we put something like "Hopeful Parent2Be". We also used one of the major email providers, again to help with anonymity. This email address was used to contact donors and join donor web sites only, and was cancelled when Sarah reached her second trimester.

Join a Sperm Donor Web Site – The easiest way to describe these sites is like a dating site for your prospective child. You enter hair color, eye color, IQ, location, and other characteristics that you would like your donor to have, and the sites bring up a profile of a man who fits those details. Typically, you need to pay a monthly membership fee to these sites. Given the fact that we knew Sarah was healthy and could probably get pregnant quickly, we decided to go with month-to-month membership, rather than prepaying a large fee in advance to cover a longer subscription period. While you could save money over time, we didn't plan on needing the services of the site for very long.

We used two web sites during our process: Sperm Donors Worldwide (also known as FSDW or DIY Baby), and Pride Angel . FSDW has a larger database, as it covers the world. Pride Angel is smaller, and specifically targets gay and lesbian families (although it's not required you be one to join). Each has their up and down sides, as well as costs associated with them.

Get In Touch With Your Prospective Donor – We learned from friends of ours to let the donor know right off the bat what your expectations are. Give them an idea of how many times per month you are looking to obtain sperm from them. Ask them if they are willing to answer additional questions (if you have them). Let them know how much contact you are willing to have with them in the event of a successful insemination. Find out their expectations of the process.

If they don't answer the questions in a way that makes you comfortable, move onto another donor. There's no need to get hung up on a single profile, as there are always other men willing to help. Don't fall into the trap that some couples find themselves in that they put themselves as the mercy of their donor. You take control of the situation right away, and lay out the ground work as to what will happen. It may sound harsh, but control is key in this process.

Create a Contract – There are a number of resources online where you can find donor contracts. One thing to keep in mind that in 99.9% of the circumstances, these contracts are not legally binding. What they do, though, is outline in writing both side's expectations, as well as provide a document that can be given to others in the event that there are any legal issues along the way (as it shows the intentions of the donor and their involvement, or lack thereof). The contract we used was based on the one at KnownDonor.com, with modifications made to suit our needs. These are referred to as 'known donor' contracts, as technically, you will meet your donor – a circumstance that doesn't happen when using a sperm bank or other completely anonymous method.

Get Them Checked Out – We also asked all our potential donors if they would be willing to be tested for STDs and STIs prior to insemination. If you think about it, a donation is unprotected sex without the sex. You are still open to various sexually transmitted diseases such as AIDS, hepatitis, and chlamydia. While there are a few places that will provide these type of tests for free or at a very low cost (Planned Parenthood for one), be prepared to offer to pay for the test if you live in an area where the donor will be required to pay out of his own pocket. Typically, these blood tests will not cost more than $70.

Meet your Donor - This is where our experiences took two paths. For the first donor we planned on using, we went through an interview process with them. We met them at a neutral location, had a bit of an interview, and arranged to meet a month later to start the process rolling. Our personal opinion was that this was a waste of time and money for us (as we drove to meet them near their hometown, which was a few hours' drive away).

Our second donor was of the mind-set that since there would not be any involvement with him, there was no need to 'get to know' him. Meeting our second donor for the first time consisted of a thirty second conversation outside a theatre in a major metropolitan area, exchanging our empty vial for his vial containing his deposit, and confirming the meet up time for the next day. The second meeting was even less – just the exchange of vials.

Make Sure the Swimmers are Ready – Ask your donor to refrain from ejaculation for at least five days before your first insemination date. That way, he has enough sperm stored up so that your first attempt has the highest chances of success. Also request that he wears loose fitting underwear, as those tighty-whiteys will keep his testes closer to his body and increase the temperature in his scrotum. Sperm survive best at a temperature slightly lower than the body – 94'F, so boxers are truly ideal.

Arrange the Deposit and Pickup – Decide how you plan on obtaining the 'goods' – that little vial of magic that will hopefully make you a baby. There are a number of ways you can go about this. For the first donor we used, we had travelled quite a bit, and were staying in a hotel room the weekend Sarah was ovulating. Our donor arrived at our hotel, we handed them a vial, and left them to do their bit in our room. When they were done, they met us down in the lobby to let us know they had finished, and we returned back to the room to start the insemination process.

he other way that you can receive your deposit somewhat resembles a drug deal. With our second donor, we met outside at a public place, after the donor had done his thing at his own home. He passed Sarah a vial of semen, she in turn gave him an empty vial for the next round. Sarah kept the vial at body temperature by placing it in her bra, between her breasts, and we returned to our home to complete the insemination there. If you are more likely to go this route, it is imperative that you move warmly and quickly. You need to keep the sperm at body temperature to preserve as many of the swimmers as possible. You also need to move quickly – sperm starts to die off in less than two hours outside the body.

Making the Magic Happen – The Insemination

One of the more frequent questions that we were asked by friends who wanted to get pregnant was how often do you try? How many attempts to do make? When do you time the attempts?

We decided that we would try for three days, with the first day being one day before ovulation, and the next two days after that. We timed the inseminations around 24 hours apart, to give the donor a chance to build his stores back up.

So now that you have your deposit, what do you do with it? We used two methods of insemination – one using a syringe, the other using a disposable menstrual cup.

Syringe Method – this is the one that instantly springs to mind when you think of at-home inseminations. No, we aren't using a turkey baster, but that's the general idea of how it works. This method is suitable if you have a few hours for the recipient to lie on her back with her butt in the air. We used these items in our attempts with the syringe method:

• Conceive Plus Conception Friendly Lubricant
• 12ml Syringes without Needles

After receiving the vial of semen, we added approximately 1tsp of lubricant to the deposit, so that there was a bit more substance to put into the syringe. This will also help the little swimmers have a bit more to swim through. We put the tip of the syringe into the vial, and slowly, as to not get any air in the syringe, lifted the plunger to get the contents of the vial into the syringe.

We made sure that the area that Sarah was laying in had everything she needed, so that she didn't need to move for a few hours – a drink, a snack, the remote control, her mobile phone, etc. She also made sure to use the bathroom beforehand, but was careful not to wipe away too much of her CM. If you are a single woman doing this on your own, you really need to be sure that you are in a spot where you won't need to get up for a couple of hours. If you are worried about potential issues (the cat needs to be let out, you're due to a package delivery, etc.) enlist a close friend to be there while you're indisposed.

With her laying on her back and a pillow under her hips, Emma slowly inserted the syringe, and pushed it so that it was as close to Sarah's cervix as possible. Again, with a slow and careful motion, Emma pushed down the plunger to empty the syringe. She left it in Sarah's body for a few minutes to be sure that the contents had a chance to 'settle' in Sarah's body. Some sites we read suggested that the woman at the receiving end try and orgasm to help the sperm travel up into her body. Unfortunately, in slightly stressful and awkward times like this, it's not always the easiest thing to do! Emma carefully removed the syringe and threw it away.

You will get some spill-out when you remove the syringe. A small vacuum is created, which pulls out some of the semen-lubricant mixture out of the body. Over the course of the next few hours, you will also get a bit dripping out as well. We placed a towel over the pillow and below Sarah's legs fore she lay down, which helped with clean-up. She also wore a menstrual pad on her panties to ck up any drips that came out for the remainder of the day.

Menstrual Cup Method – This method is better for those who don't have the luxury of lying down for a few hours. We also feel that this method gives you a bit of an edge, as when you use the cup, you don't get the drips and spills that you get with the syringe method. It also leaves the semen 'secured' into place for a longer period of time. The down side to this method that you have to fumble a bit with the cup, which can be a bit tricky if you have never used these types of menstrual cups before. Sarah practiced a few months in advance, and used them for her period to get used to insertion. It's also quite difficult for the partner to be involved in this insemination process, since it's easier for a woman to insert the cup herself rather than have a partner do it.

In order to inseminate via the menstrual cup method, you'll need a couple of items.

• Conceive Plus Conception Friendly Lubricant
• Instead Softcups – you want to use a soft type menstrual cup, not the more firm cups like the Diva Cup or the Moon Cup.

After you've received your deposit, you open up one of the softcups and pour in about 1tsp of lubricant. You then tip the contents of your vial into the cup. This is where it gets a bit tricky and messy. You need to squeeze the cup to insert it into your body, but you want to be careful as not lose any of the liquid inside of it. Once it is secured into place, you can go about your business. No need to lay down, since the cup holds the contents against your cervix.

Sarah inserted hers in the late afternoon, and left it in overnight. In the morning she removed the cup and threw it into the garbage.

Part Two – Our Story : From Our First Attempts to a Positive Pregnancy Test

this part, we present our story as a whole. This means that some information that we have scussed in the previous sections may be repeated, but we feel it's important to keep the entire story context.

'e decided to wait until we had purchased our first home before trying to have a baby. It had been ell established beforehand that Sarah would be the one to conceive, as Emma didn't have any esire at all to go through insemination and pregnancy. We also decided that we did not want to ave any involvement with our donor following a successful insemination. This meant that we would ot make the donor aware that Sarah was pregnant. A month after we moved into our home, Sarah arted taking prenatal vitamins, and started weaning herself of medication that would have a egative effect on a fetus.

uring this time, we discovered and joined Sperm Donors Worldwide. As had been suggested by a ndom website online, we made our anonymous email address. It took us around six weeks to ade through the profiles of men in the part of the UK that we live in, and narrow it down to a lection of four or five that we contacted. Sarah handled most of the interactions between the nors and ourselves. In her first email out to prospective donors, she asked a series of questions, cluding:

- Have you ever donated to lesbian couples before?
- If you have, how many successful inseminations are you aware of?
- Do you have your own children? [We ask this question to gauge the possible issue of having donor contact after insemination is successful.]
- Is your partner aware of your desire to assist us with our insemination? If so, what are their thoughts on the matter?
- Are you comfortable with having no contact with us whatsoever following a successful insemination?
- Can you provide us with a photo of yourself now, as well as a photo of you when you were under five years old?
- Can you confirm that the information related to health issues in your profile is correct?
- Can you provide STD blood tests results dated within the last six months showing that you are free from any diseases?

ce we found a man that answered the questions in ways that made us feel comfortable, we began arrange a meet up. (For the sake of the story, we'll call him Mike.) Sarah had been tracking her riods using the date tracking method, and the cervical fluid method. We made Mike aware of the 's that Sarah would be best off being inseminated.

this point, we felt that we wanted to 'get to know' the donor a bit before we actually went ough with the insemination. This was a bit difficult for us, though, as the donor we had chosen lived more than a three hour drive away. So we arranged to stay in a hotel room for 2 nights, and meet the donor at a restaurant attached to the hotel on the first evening there.

First impressions were fine, and after a bit of chit chat we went back to the room for, what we assumed, would be a quick process. Little did we know that our donor had different ideas.

Rather than leaving him in the room to do his thing, Mike wanted to chat. For two more hours. He wanted to know the ins and outs of our relationship, our likes and dislikes, our working life and a lot more. He shared with us the experiences he had with other couples and how all of the children that he produced still had contact with him. He made fun of the hobbies Emma enjoys and sarcastically mimicked Sarah's American accent. He told us about the porn that he brought with him to help him around. Red flags were going up left, right and center.

Finally, when Mike decided it was time to get the show on the road, we went downstairs into the lobby to wait for him to finish. So began a manic few moments of conversation between us. If he had acted this way while we were in the restaurant, we probably would have walked out the door and started the three hour drive back to our house. But, independently, we were questioning our decision. Had we gone too far to turn around? How long would it take us to find another donor? We had already taken months to find Mike only to have it 'wasted' now. If we did go through with it, do we really want this man to be the genetic 'father' of our child?

Before we could make a decision, Mike walked down the stairs and announced he had left his deposit. In our confused state, we agreed to meet up tomorrow for the next donation. We had arranged online to try for 3 days in a row, and with all the craziness of the last two hours, we had forgot that factor. We both just nodded in agreement and went up to the room.

When we got back to the room, it came to be decision time. Were we going to go through with this? Despite our hesitations, despite our absolute disgust in the guy that we had thought was "the one" we went for it.

With deep breaths and shaking hands, Sarah went into the bathroom and took the specimen cup. She was a bit surprised at the lack of 'stuff' in the cup, but from her research beforehand, we knew that even in the tiniest drop of semen, millions of sperm are swimming. She added a few drops of Conceive Plus into the jar, and slowly sucked it all up into the syringe.

Meanwhile, Emma was preparing the area for Sarah to lie down. She made sure that Sarah's cell phone, a drink, something to snack on, the TV remote, and her books were on the bedside table. S laid down a towel over the bed to avoid any 'wet spots' when we slept there that night. She also stacked a few pillows half way down the bed, and covered those with a towel as well.

Sarah came into the room with the syringe, and left it with Emma while she went to pee. When she was done, she took off her underwear and got onto the bed. The pillows made it so that Sarah's hi were somewhat elevated, and soon the position was assumed. We took out the vibrator, as we ha heard that orgasms help guide the swimmers upward to their target, but we just about laughed ou asses off with the thought of trying to get me to cum with this whole scenario and the nerves running through the both of us.

We kissed each other, then went forward with the plan. Slowly Emma inserted the syringe into Sarah, and pressed down on the plunger. A bit of the mixture of semen and lube came out the sides, so Emma started to panic slightly. She readjusted the syringe, pushed it in a bit further, and emptied out the entire contents. We left the syringe in there for about twenty minutes. When that time was up, Emma pulled it out and threw it away. We still had more 'spillage', but we knew at that point, we did the best we could. The next few hours Sarah stayed in that position, and just let the magic happen. After the time had passed, Sarah showered , put on a menstrual pad, and we went out for dinner.

The next two days with Mike were unfortunately very much the same. Hours of awkward chit chat, followed by ten minutes waiting in the lobby for him to finish. We went through the same steps as the first day, hoping that we wouldn't have to go through this process again.

Unfortunately, a negative pregnancy test two weeks later let us know that we would have to do this again. We arranged with Mike to try again next month, and let him know a few days in advance which days would be best. Sarah started using the ferning and basal body temperature methods to track her periods in addition to the date and CM that she had already started. Based on this new information we selected another 3 days of insemination, made Mike aware, and booked the hotel room.

Mike was the same as the previous meetings – trying to be overly friendly and insulting all at the same time. We went through three days of inseminations, but were once again faced with a negative pregnancy test.

Problems with our families started to become more and more difficult to handle after this second insemination attempt. So much that Sarah's periods skipped, and her cycle was thrown for a loop. The patterns and times that we had worked so hard to track were now completely unpredictable. It took about 3 months for them to return to normal, and during this time we didn't speak much with Mike, save letting him know that we wouldn't be trying that month.

The conversation, though, made it clear to us that Mike was no longer someone we wanted to have in our lives, even for a temporary time.

The last time we spoke with him, he made us aware that he was starting to have intercourse with one of the other couples that he was trying to help. He let us know that they had been using the 'usual' methods for months with no success and now they were just going to start having sex. He noted that this was something we should be looking at.

Not only were we not aware that Mike was actively working with other couples (and possibly reducing his sperm count for our sessions), the fact that he was even fathoming having sex with Sarah was something we didn't want to even discuss. We made it clear to Mike that we were not happy with this arrangement, and that we would be looking to seek the services of another donor.

Tears came. Hours of tears, as we thought that our only opportunity was now gone. For days, Sarah moped around the house, blaming herself for not getting pregnant. She also blamed herself for not handling the family issues well enough and sending herself into stress induced period skipping. Emma did her best to console her, but she was also going through her own set of blame. Was she not doing the insemination correctly? Was she not helping Sarah deal with family issues enough? After a long series of conversations, the pity party was ended, and a new day began.

We started from scratch.

Sarah purchased a Clear Blue Easy Fertility Monitor and started using it at the start of her next cycle. We also decided that we would try the menstrual cup method this time, and leave the syringes behind.

Pride Angels was a site we learned about at a trip to the local Pride event. It was a donor site that was just starting out, and specifically tailored to gay families. Not only was it a sperm donor directory, it was a surrogate and co-parenting search site. We joined, and once again narrowed it down to a few new donors. Ironically, Mike had also discover this site, as we found a profile that wa a duplicate of his on Sperm Donors Worldwide.

We found a donor (who we'll call Drew) who lived less than an hour away. Technically, we could tak the donation and bring it back to our house for insemination. Unfortunately, Sarah's fertile periods covered a Sunday, Monday and Tuesday. After discussions with Drew, we decided to try just two days – the Sunday and the Monday.

This time, there would be no chit chat. We arranged to meet Drew in a very public park in the midd of the city. From the outside, it must have looked like a drug deal. Drew came up to us and confirmed the fake names we had given him. He handed Sarah a vial filled with his semen, and she handed him an empty one in return. She placed the vial between her breasts, zipped up her jacket against the cold February winter, and we walked back to our awaiting car.

When we arrived home, Sarah held the Instead Cup open while Emma poured in the liquid from the vial. We added a few drops of Conceive Plus, then inserted it into Sarah's body. She had been using the cup while we were waiting for her to get regular again, so there was no issue with getting it in correctly. She propped up her legs on the side of the couch, and we watched a few movies to pass the time. The next day, the process was repeated again.

Two weeks later, Sarah woke before Emma and did the classic pee-on-a-stick pregnancy test. After the two minute waiting time, no line appeared. With tears in her eyes, she left it on the bedside table where she brought it while it 'developed', and took a shower. A bleary eyed Emma met Sarah in the hallway and they exchanged kisses while Emma went in to take her shower.

Sarah went back to the bedroom, and picked up the test to throw in the trash. Having a second loo at it, she noticed a second line had appeared. It was faint, but it was certainly there.

Sarah was pregnant.

We kept taking pregnancy tests every day for the next week, just to be sure that it was true. Famili were told the news, and later on in the pregnancy friends were made aware. On November 3rd, 2010, our son Thomas was born through a natural water birth here in England. We have never bee happier.

When we made others aware that we were pregnant, that's when the questions started. First, we had a few single mom friends who wanted to have babies without dealing with sperm banks and o ght stands. Then we had lesbian friends who asked us how we did it. Then it was friends of friends no were embarrassed they were asking perfect strangers how they got knocked up, but were sperate to have babies of their own. On average we got asked at least once every six weeks how e did it – and now we've written a book to help those like us to successfully become pregnant on a dget.

Acknowledgements and Contact Info

We'd like to thank a few folks for their help with this book.

Sarah's family for being completely supportive throughout the whole process – including the pregnancy.

Our friends for putting up with the FB updates, especially the editing circle ('Itchy' Jen, 'Sunshine' Alicia, Kara, Erin, Lou, Jessie, Jody and Heather) who volunteered their time to check through the various forms of this book. Especially to her sister-in-law Jess for being her 'pregnancy mirror' for nine months (less a few weeks at the end).

For the numerous lesbian couples who pushed us to write a book based on our own experiences and those that smacked us on the back of the head when we missed out on writing a follow up for single mothers and heterosexual couples.

And of course, our little man Thomas who was the whole reason for this book's existence.

...

We ask that you kindly review this book once you have read it. Your comments will be taken into consideration when publishing further editions.

If you are interested in finding out more about the products and services we have mentioned here please join us at http://lesbian-mothers.com . While the website is designed for same sex mothers we discuss all the products featured here, along with many more that will assist you in achieving a natural pregnancy.

Printed in Great Britain
by Amazon